Pneumonia

Simon Godfrey, MD, PhD, FRCP
Professor of Paediatrics
Director, Institute of Pulmonology
Hadassah University Hospital
Jerusalem, Israel

Robert Wilson, MD, FRCP
Consultant Physician and Senior Lecturer
Host Defence Unit
Royal Brompton Hospital and National
Heart and Lung Institute
London, UK

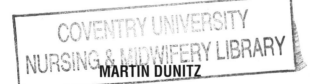
MARTIN DUNITZ

Coventry University

© Martin Dunitz Ltd 1996

First published in the United Kingdom
in 1996 by
Martin Dunitz Ltd
The Livery House
7– 9 Pratt Street
London NW1 0AE

A CIP record for this book is available
from the British Library.

ISBN 1-85317-241-3

Printed and bound in Spain by Cayfosa

Po 00215

Contents

Acknowledgements

The authors wish to thank the following colleagues who have offered their advice and provided information or illustrations which have been included in the text:

Professor J Bar-Ziv, Department of Radiology, Hadassah University Hospital; Dr D Engelhard, Department of Pediatrics, Hadassah University Hospital; Dr R Breuer, Department of Pulmonology, Hadassah University Hospital; Ms Evelyn Holmes, Information Pharmacist, Royal Brompton Hospital; Dr Tony Howard, Department of Microbiology, Ysbyty Gwynedd, Bangor; and Mr Peter Webber, Royal Brompton Hospital.

However, responsibility for the text and for any errors which have inadvertently occurred is entirely that of the authors.

The authors also wish to thank their secretaries Mrs S Berger and Mrs Jane Burditt for their help in preparing the manuscript and Jacky Alderson of Martin Dunitz Ltd for all her help and encouragement.

Definition and causes of pneumonia

Respiratory infections of all kinds are extremely common causes of morbidity and mortality at all ages and are particularly dangerous in those whose resistance is weakened through prematurity or disease and in the elderly. Pneumonia ranks sixth in the leading causes of death and ranks even higher in the aged. It is the third commonest hospital-acquired infection and the incidence of pneumonia is increasing as new predisposing factors are appearing. These include the emergence of resistant strains of organisms and the increase in the immunocompromised population through disease such as human immunodeficiency virus (HIV) infection, treatment of malignancies and treatment for the purpose of organ transplantation.

Pneumonia refers specifically to an inflammatory disease process involving the lung parenchyma rather than disease of the conducting airways, although both may occur at the same time. While by far the commonest cause of pneumonia is invasion of the lungs by a micro-organism, other non-infective processes can also cause alveolar or interstitial inflammation. Pneumonia may be classified according to the source of infection, the infectious agent or the major site of the pathological process. Treatment is often commenced on an empirical basis and changed if necessary when the results of investigations become available. The choice of empirical treatment will be influenced by knowledge of the most likely infectious agent in any given set of circumstances and by its likely antimicrobial susceptibility. In this book the clinical manifestations, investigation and treatment of infective pneumonias are considered. The non-infective pneumonias form a quite distinctive group of diseases and will not be discussed in detail in the sections which follow.

Classification of pneumonia

By source of infection

Community-acquired	• Pneumococcal pneumonia most common in adults • *Haemophilus* pneumonia very common in children • *Mycoplasma* pneumonia common in both (epidemics occur every 3–4 years)
Hospital-acquired or nosocomial	• Increased incidence of Gram-negative bacterial infections • Higher mortality than with community-acquired infections • Underlying condition of patient important in prognosis
Aspiration of foreign material	• More common in infancy and childhood • May cause chemical pneumonitis • Anaerobic bacteria likely in adults, less so in children • May be unsuspected in the elderly
The immuno-compromised host	• Wide range of micro-organisms, including those of normally low pathogenicity • May rapidly become life-threatening because of absence of host defences • Often require invasive diagnostic procedures to identify infectious agent

By infectious agent

Bacterial pneumonia	• Common at all ages • Many organisms can cause pneumonia in healthy subjects • Some bacteria have a tendency to attack susceptible subjects, e.g. *Klebsiella* in the alcoholic person or *Staphylococcus* after an influenza viral infection • Most bacterial pneumonias are curable by appropriate medication
Atypical pneumonia	• Due to *Mycoplasma, Legionella, Chlamydia, Coxiella* • The older child and young adult are most commonly affected • Require a macrolide or tetracycline and do not respond to beta-lactam antibiotics
Viral pneumonia	• More common in infants and children • More likely to be serious in subjects with weakened resistance • Some viral pneumonias are susceptible to medication
Fungi and other infective agents	• Often represent secondary infection • Predilection for debilitated patients • May attack healthy subjects and some are endemic • Treatment can be problematic

By site of infection

The pathological classification of pneumonia by site has lost much of its significance as far as lobar and bronchopneumonia are concerned. Most organisms can cause both forms of the disease and the extent of the pneumonia depends upon various host factors and the appropriateness and speed with which treatment is given.

Lobar pneumonia (Fig. 1)	• More common in bacterial pneumonia
	• Less common in infancy and the elderly
	• Pneumonia localized to a lobe or segment may be secondary to obstruction of the supplying bronchus and this should always be considered if the clinical setting is appropriate, e.g. foreign body aspiration in a child or malignancy in an adult
Broncho-pneumonia (Fig. 2)	• Patchy and widespread throughout lungs
	• Can be due to bacteria as well as viruses
	• Common in infancy and the elderly
	• Unlikely to be associated with bronchial obstruction
Interstitial pneumonia (Fig. 3)	• Involves interstitium rather than alveoli or bronchi
	• Characteristic radiological changes on plain film or CT scan
	• Typical of opportunistic infection (cytomegalovirus, *Pneumocystis carinii*)
	• Typical of non-infective pneumonias

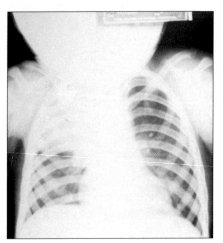

Figure 1
Lobar pneumonia due to Strep. pneumoniae in the right upper lobe of a child.

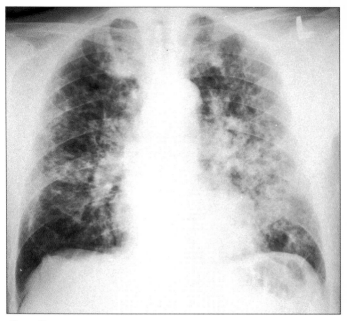

Figure 2
Bronchopneumonia with bilateral irregular patchy infiltrates in an adult.

Non-infective pneumonia

This category includes interstitial diseases of unknown origin such as fibrosing alveolitis and its various pathological subdivisions, e.g. desquamative interstitial pneumonia, usual interstitial pneumonia and lymphocytic interstitial pneumonitis (often associated with HIV infection); eosinophilic pneumonias either confined to the lung or associated with systemic disease such as the Churg–Strauss syndrome; bronchiolitis obliterans with organizing pneumonia (BOOP), also called cryptogenic organizing pneumonia (COP), which may be a primary lung disease or associated with multisystem diseases; and chemical pneumonitis, e.g. smoke inhalation, toxic gas inhalation, aspiration syndromes.

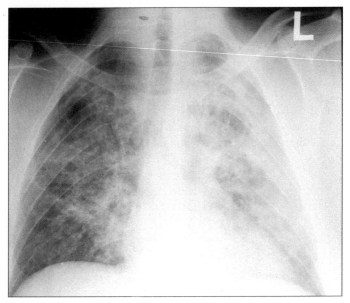

Figure 3
Interstitial pneumonia more marked on the left with diffuse interstitial markings due to Pneumocystis carinii infection in a patient with AIDS.

Susceptibility to pneumonia

The organisms which cause infective pneumonia are very numerous and most are found in large numbers in the air we breathe and in the food we eat; they often live with us as commensals without causing any trouble. The lungs are continuously exposed to the environment, and the reason why they are not continuously infected lies with the natural defence mechanisms of the body.

Filtration of inspired air in the nose and upper airways, cough and mucociliary transport all remove foreign material from the respiratory system. Invading organisms may be dealt with in a number of ways including non-specific antibacterial activity, e.g. surfactant and factors in mucus such as lysozyme, and phagocytosis by polymorphonuclear leukocytes and alveolar macrophages. Organisms may also be opsonized by complement or by local and systemic immunoglobulins; it is also possible for complement to destroy them directly. Finally, the presence of specific immunoglobulins and IgA, activation of cell-mediated immunity and cytokine secretion are all important factors in protecting the lungs from infective agents.

Under certain circumstances these mechanisms fail and allow organisms to get past the defences and cause pneumonia. Often there is no obvious reason for this susceptibility in healthy subjects exposed to a causative agent, e.g. pneumococcal pneumonia or tuberculosis in a healthy adult. A large dose of the infecting agent, unusual virulence of the microorganism, recent viral infection, or lack of host immunity to a particular strain are all possible factors contributing to infection. More obvious predisposing factors include:

- Bronchial obstruction which prevents the free drainage of secretions, e.g. congenital anomaly of the airway (bronchomalacia), foreign body impaction, mucus plugging or bronchial carcinoma

- Aspiration of food or fluids, e.g. unconscious subjects, gastro-oesophageal reflux, tracheo-oesophageal fistula, neurological disease

- Abnormalities of normal mucociliary clearance, e.g. weak cough, chronic bronchitis, cystic fibrosis, primary ciliary dyskinesia (immotile cilia) syndrome

- Endotracheal intubation, ventilation or instrumentation of airway, all of which can damage normal defence mechanisms and expose lungs to upper airway flora

- Humoral or cellular immunodeficiency, e.g. HIV infection, severe combined immunodeficiency (SCID) of infancy, chemotherapy for malignant disease or immunosuppression following organ transplantation

- Environmental factors such as an infected water supply (*Legionella*) or infected birds (Psittacosis)

- Splenectomy and sickle-cell disease causing splenic infarction and producing functional splenectomy. These patients are specifically sensitive to pneumococcal infection.

True immunodeficiency, even in the age of HIV infection, is a rare cause of pneumonia in the general population. However, a high index of suspicion of a host defence problem is recommended if pneumonia occurs repeatedly.

Finally, the very young, the very old and debilitated subjects without overt immunodeficiency are all susceptible to pneumonia.

The prevention of pneumonia

Having considered the defence mechanisms available and the reasons why these may be overwhelmed, we should now consider what, if any, steps can be taken to prevent patients from catching pneumonia.

Avoidance of exposure to infection

Public health measures to prevent overcrowding and improvement in social conditions are both fundamental to the prevention of pneumonia. Infectious individuals, especially patients with tuberculosis, should be isolated and treated.

Immunization of susceptible populations

Pneumococcal immunization for splenectomized patients is advisable; the benefits in the older population and in patients with chronic lung disease are less certain. Infants are now being immunized against *Haemophilus influenzae* type B as a cause of meningitis and it remains to be seen how this will affect susceptibility to pneumonia. Patients with chronic lung diseases should receive immunization against relevant strains of influenza viruses before each winter. Finally, BCG immunization reduces the risk of tuberculosis although studies in different countries have shown variable benefit.

Prevention of hospital-acquired infections

This can be achieved by careful attention to nursing techniques, especially in intubated patients, and careful attention to the avoidance of cross-infection in patients at risk, especially immunocompromised patients of all types.

Prevention of aspiration of foreign material

This can be achieved by attention to the airway of unconscious subjects; forbidding the eating of peanuts and other small nuts by young children; and proper management of gastro-oesophageal reflux.

Removal of retained secretions

This involves regular physiotherapy and postural drainage for patients with defective lung clearance mechanisms or chronic suppurative lung diseases, e.g. bronchiectasis.

Organisms most likely to cause pneumonia in specific patient groups

A list of the organisms which may be found in patients with pneumonia under different circumstances is given in Appendix A.

In the newborn

The commonest pathogens in the first 3 months of life are respiratory viruses, especially respiratory syncytial virus (RSV), but also adenovirus, influenza and parainfluenza viruses. Non-respiratory viruses are also important at this age, including cytomegalovirus (CMV), enteroviruses and Herpes simplex.

In the immediate postnatal period an early onset of pneumonia, within 48 h after birth, is commoner with prolonged rupture of the membranes, and the likeliest pathogen is Group B *Streptococcus*, which may be rapidly fatal if untreated.

After 2–3 weeks, *Chlamydia* is a possible cause of pneumonia, especially if the infant has signs of an eye infection or the mother has a vaginal discharge.

In the neonatal intensive care nursery, nosocomial infections with *Staphylococcus aureus*, *Escherichia coli*, *Pseudomonas aeruginosa*, *Serratia marcescens*, *Klebsiella*, streptococci and sometimes *Candida* are all recognized, and the likeliest organism varies from nursery to nursery.

In the younger child

Respiratory viruses are the most common pathogens causing pneumonia in the infant and young child. Bacterial pneumonia in small children is most commonly due to *Haemophilus influenzae* even in those in whom there is an underlying problem of aspiration. Pneumococcal infections are less likely and *Mycoplasma* infection usually occurs in older children. Opportunistic infections such as those due to *Pneumocystis carinii* suggest immunodeficiency and may be the presenting feature of HIV infection in early childhood.

Pneumonia due to *Staphylococcus aureus, E. coli* or *P. aeruginosa* is uncommon in early childhood but is found in children with immunodeficiency and cystic fibrosis.

In the older child and adult

Pneumococcus, H. influenzae and *Mycoplasma* are the most common pathogens in the older child and adult. *Mycoplasma* epidemics occur about every 4 years. Influenza virus is the most common viral pathogen, usually but not always with secondary bacterial infection. Post-influenza staphylococcal pneumonia has high mortality but is rare.

Gram-negative infections (apart from those due to *H. influenzae*) are uncommon in the community in the UK, but are more commonly reported in the US.

In the elderly

Pneumococcus is the most common pathogen in the elderly. *Mycoplasma* infections are uncommon.

Nursing home studies show an increase in the incidence of Gram-negative pneumonias which probably relates to frequent use of antibiotics, silent aspiration, crowded care and reduction in the host defences with age.

In the immunocompromised host

Numerous organisms may cause pneumonia in the immuno-compromised host, as follows:

Bacteria	*Streptococcus pneumoniae; Streptococcus spp.; Haemophilus influenzae;* Gram-negative bacilli; environmental mycobacteria, e.g. *Mycobacterium avium-intracellulare; Nocardia asteroides*
Fungi	*Aspergillus spp.; Cryptococcus neoformans; Pneumocystis carinii*
Viruses	Cytomegalovirus
Parasites	*Strongyloides stercoralis*

After bone marrow or organ transplantation, early pneumonia is usually bacterial or fungal (*Candida, Aspergillus*); pneumonia within 1–2 months is often due to *Pneumocystis carinii* unless the patient is receiving prophylaxis; and pneumonia after 2–4 months is often due to cytomegalovirus.

HIV-related pneumonia may be bacterial, viral or (non-infective) lymphocytic interstitial pneumonitis. Tuberculosis is a common infection.

Clinical presentation of pneumonia

Classically, pneumonia presents as an acute febrile illness with cough, dyspnoea and sputum production and with signs of consolidation. However, this picture is only typical of some types of bacterial pneumonia in an otherwise healthy subject. A recent summary of community-acquired pneumonia produced for the American Thoracic Society stressed the poor value of the history, physical examination, routine laboratory tests and radiological examination in predicting the likely pathogen. Amongst the factors influencing the clinical picture are the age of the patient, the presence of other complicating illnesses and the nature of the infecting organism.

Clinical features of pneumonia in particular patient groups

In the newborn

The clinical features of pneumonia in the newborn are non-specific and common to other causes of sepsis; correct diagnosis can often only be made with the help of radiological and other ancillary investigations. The features are:

- Poor sucking, refusal to feed, lethargy, hypotonia
- Recurring apnoeic spells, prolonged apnoea
- Hypoxia, increased requirements for added inspired oxygen
- Hypothermia or hyperthermia
- Tachypnoea and tachycardia
- Respiratory distress is less obvious than in older infants
- Physical examination is relatively unhelpful
- Thrombocytopenia, leukopenia or leukocytosis

Always consider the possibility of: meningitis and other types of sepsis; heart failure; intraventricular haemorrhage; and necrotizing enterocolitis in the premature infant.

In the infant and young child

The clinical features of pneumonia are more obvious in the infant and young child than in the newborn, although the symptoms and signs are affected by the young age of the patient. The features are:

- Tachypnoea
- Nasal flaring
- Fever
- Cough
- May present with abdominal pain
- Small children swallow their sputum and the cough is rarely productive
- Refusal to eat
- Wheezing is common with viral pneumonia and also with gastro-oesophageal reflux and aspiration
- Physical examination – bronchopneumonia common and crepitations often heard bilaterally
- Leukocytosis common but not essential
- Extrapulmonary signs of infection may also be present – otitis media, sinusitis, conjunctivitis, meningitis

Always consider the possibility of: other sites of infection (especially abdominal); foreign body aspiration; cystic fibrosis; gastro-oesophageal reflux and aspiration.

In the older child or adult

The clinical features of pneumonia in the older child or adult are:

- Fever – possibly rigors
- Myalgia, arthralgia, headache
- Cough
- Sputum production – as a new symptom or with a change in the quantity or colour in patients with chronic bronchitis
- Dyspnoea
- Haemoptysis – beware of malignancy underlying pneumonia
- Pleuritic pain, which may radiate to the abdomen or tip of the shoulder
- On physical examination – signs of consolidation in lobar pneumonia, e.g. bronchial breathing, dullness to percussion, increased vocal fremitus, localized crepitations; diffuse crepitations in bronchopneumonia
- Herpes labialis (especially with pneumococcal pneumonia)
- Stony dullness to percussion with reduced breath sounds and absent vocal fremitus suggests pleural effusion
- May be discrepancy between paucity of physical signs and marked radiographic changes in *Mycoplasma* pneumonia
- Leukocytosis is usual, except in viral or *Mycoplasma* pneumonia

Always consider: other sites of infection, especially abdominal emergencies; a host defence problem if pneumonia is recurrent.

In the elderly

There is often a paucity of symptoms and signs of pneumonia in the elderly, however the following clinical features may be seen:

- Tachypnoea
- Dyspnoea, laboured breathing
- Cough with or without sputum production
- Haemoptysis – beware underlying malignancy
- Mental confusion and deterioration in general condition
- Fever not always present – may be only a little elevated
- On physical examination – signs of bronchopneumonia are commoner than those of lobar pneumonia. May be signs of pleural fluid or signs of congestive cardiac failure

Always consider the possibility of: malignancy underlying pneumonia; heart failure as alternative diagnosis or secondary to pneumonia; and ischaemic heart disease as a cause of chest pain and respiratory distress in the elderly patient.

In the immunocompromised host

The clinical features of pneumonia in the immunocompromised host include:

- Possible presentation as apparently uncomplicated but recurrent pneumonia

- Often insidious onset of dry cough, progressive dyspnoea, tachypnoea and hypoxia

- Fever is an important clue in many patients

- New lesions on the chest radiograph may be the only feature

- Blood picture depends upon underlying disease

- May give a history of infections at other sites

- May present as unexplained bronchiectasis

- May occur after bone marrow or solid organ transplantation

- HIV-related pneumonia may be bacterial, viral or (non-infective) lymphocytic interstitial pneumonitis. Tuberculosis is a common pathogen where the two diseases coexist.

Always consider: a wide range of possible pathogens – virulent and opportunistic organisms; viral, fungal and tuberculous infections; non-infective processes, which can cause pulmonary infiltrates.

In patients who have aspirated infected material

The clinical features of pneumonia in patients who have aspirated infected material include:

- Possible history of choking on food, but absence of a history does not exclude diagnosis

- Sudden onset of cough/dyspnoea in a previously healthy young child suggests foreign body aspiration. Peak age is 1–3 years.

- Recurrent chest infections, often with wheezing and failure to thrive, suggests gastro-oesophageal reflux and aspiration in an infant or young child

- Recurrent chest infections from early infancy may suggest a congenital anomaly connecting the airway and oesophagus (very rare). Oesophageal atresia presents within minutes of birth

- Atelectasis or localized hyperinflation of recent onset on the chest radiograph is suggestive of foreign body aspiration in a patient with a compatible history

- Haemoptysis in an otherwise healthy child or young adult suggests aspiration

- Onset of cough, fever and sputum production after a period of unconsciousness suggests aspiration and possibly the development of a lung abscess. The organism may be an anaerobe

- Disorders of oesophageal motility and gastro-oesophageal reflux in the adult (particularly the elderly) may result in recurrent aspiration pneumonia

- Acid aspiration may cause pulmonary oedema

- With anaerobic infections there may be necrotizing pneumonia (multiple small abscesses usually in more than one lobe); larger lung abscess or empyema are common complications

Always consider: deficiency in swallowing mechanism and neurological disorders.

Clinical features of pneumonia due to particular organisms

Atypical pneumonia

This is most common in adolescents and younger adults. It has a more gradual onset than a typical pneumonia, often beginning with sore throat or earache. A dry cough and profound systemic symptoms are also clinical features. Often all members of the family are infected but with different severity, ranging from asymptomatic to severely ill with pneumonia.

Atypical pneumonia should always be considered as a possibility, since it is impossible to judge the infecting micro-organism from clinical features alone.

Tuberculosis

Until recently the incidence of tuberculosis (TB) had steadily declined in the developed world, but there has been a resurgence of the disease, and multi-drug-resistant TB is increasing worldwide (although not so far in the UK). Inhalation is the most important mode of transmission.

Primary TB is usually self-contained with no symptoms, but progressive destructive lung disease occurs in a few patients. Secondary or reactivation TB occurs years later as upper lobe pneumonia. Apical scars on the lungs, old age, alcoholism, diabetes, silicosis, prolonged steroid treatment and malignancy increase the risk of reactivation of TB.

Common symptoms of TB are cough, haemoptysis, fever, malaise, night sweats and weight loss. Massive enlargement of mediastinal lymph nodes may cause severe large airway obstruction.

TB should always be considered – it is correctly described as the great mimic because of its variable clinical presentation.

Environmental (atypical) mycobacterial infection

This is usually a secondary infection in damaged lungs, e.g. bronchiectasis, bullae, old scarred TB. *M. avium-intracellulare* especially can cause primary disease and is a common lung pathogen in AIDS.

Environmental mycobacterial infection can present like TB, or as deterioration of a chronic condition. It is difficult to treat because of antibiotic resistance.

Virus pneumonia

Virus pneumonia is a potentially lethal complication of influenza, with cough, dyspnoea and cyanosis developing as part of the influenza illness.The chest radiograph shows diffuse progressive bilateral infiltrates.

Herpes virus infections (cytomegalovirus and Herpes simplex) occur in immunocompromised patients and varicella pneumonia may occur in young adults, although it is rare in childhood.

Secondary bacterial infection should always be considered, especially in patients with increased risk, e.g. chronic lung disease, diabetes, or heart disease. Such patients should receive influenza vaccine before the winter epidemic.

Fungus pneumonia

Primary fungal infections, e.g. coccidioidomycosis, histoplasmosis and blastomycosis, occur in healthy individuals in particular geographical areas, e.g. North America, and most infections are mild. Fungal infections occur more commonly in the immunocompromised patient.

Allergic bronchopulmonary aspergillosis (ABPA) occurs in association with asthma, but can occur in non-asthmatic individuals and in cystic fibrosis. The features of ABPA include fleeting shadows on chest radiograph due to eosinophilic infiltration, mucus plugs with atelectasis, blood eosinophilia, positive skin test, serum precipitins or positive radioallergosorbent (RAST) tests, elevated IgE and fungus grown in sputum.

Fungal infection should always be considered in the immuno-compromised patient and ABPA in the difficult asthmatic patient.

Pneumocystis carinii pneumonia

This occurs in up to 80% of AIDS cases and may have an insidious onset. The clinical features are a dry cough, dyspnoea and fever. Bilateral perihilar haze may be seen on chest radiograph, but up to 10% of symptomatic patients have normal radiographs. Hypoxaemia is a common feature and reflects the severity of the pneumonitis.

Clinical improvement is commonly delayed for 5 to 7 days after starting treatment, and patients may actually deteriorate during the first couple of days.

It is important to consider that immunosuppressed patients may harbour more than one pathogen causing the infection.

Features suggestive of an uncommon organism causing pneumonia

There are several features that may suggest that an uncommon organism is responsible for pneumonia in a patient. There may be a failure to respond to antibiotic therapy appropriate for the most likely bacterial pathogens or a discrepancy between the chest radiograph and the clinical condition.

Severe obstructive lung disease in infants and children is commonly associated with viral infections and severe systemic involvement, abnormal liver function, and thrombocytopenia in these patients are often associated with adenoviral infection.

Legionella infections are commonly associated with severe systemic, gastrointestinal and neurological symptoms.

Elderly or debilitated patients are susceptible to *Klebsiella* and other Gram-negative bacteria and immunocompromised and HIV-infected patients are susceptible to various uncommon pathogens. Patients with cystic fibrosis are often infected by *Pseudomonas* or *Staph. aureus* and patients with aspiration pneumonia may be infected with anaerobic organisms or *Actinomyces.*

Tuberculosis is still very common in many parts of the world and should always be considered in the diagnosis of unresolving pneumonia. If the patient is not responding to treatment always consider the following:

- That the patient has not been taking the prescribed treatment
- That the dose or route of administration of medication was inappropriate
- That the infecting organism was not correctly identified
- That the patient has developed a complication, e.g. empyema or metastatic abscess

Evaluating the likely severity of pneumonia

Given the wide variability of the clinical manifestations of pneumonia, it is impossible to define the severity of the disease in a categorical fashion, but there are a number of features which are indicative of a heightened risk of morbidity or mortality.

Pneumonia is more likely to be serious in:

- The very young and the very old and the malnourished
- Patients with concomitant chronic lung disease such as cystic fibrosis, chronic obstructive pulmonary disease (COPD) and bronchiectasis
- Patients with concomitant non-pulmonary chronic disease such as congenital heart disease, heart failure, diabetes, or liver or kidney disease
- Patients who have aspirated foreign material into the lungs
- Immunocompromised patients
- Patients who partake in alcohol or drug abuse
- Patients in whom there is a delay between the onset of disease and the beginning of treatment

- Marked tachypnoea (rate dependent on age); >30/min in adults, higher in children
- Marked hyperthermia (>40°C)
- Marked hypoxia (saturation on air < 85%)
- Systemic hypotension (level dependent on age); diastolic pressure < 60 mmHg in adults
- Mental confusion, drowsiness
- Concomitant extrapulmonary sites of infection
- Multilobar disease
- Deteriorating radiological picture with spread of the disease (can occur in infections with *Mycoplasma* and *Legionella* despite appropriate antibiotics)
- Marked leukocytosis (>30 000/mm^3) or leukopenia (< 4000/mm^3)
- Respiratory failure (high PCO_2 >45 mmHg in an adult or >40 mmHg in a child)
- Thrombocytopenia, disseminated intravascular coagulopathy, metabolic acidosis (pH < 7.3)

Pleural disease complicating pneumonia

Any pneumonic process which reaches the pleural surface may give rise to an exudate of fluid into the pleural space. In many cases the fluid remains sterile and small in volume. This type of uncomplicated effusion is termed a parapneumonic effusion. If the fluid is infected it becomes purulent and is then termed an empyema. Progression of the empyema to loculation, organization and fibrosis leading to restriction of the underlying lung may occur if an empyema is inadequately treated. Empyema used to be relatively common as a complication of pneumococcal pneumonia, but with modern treatment this is much less likely. Parapneumonic effusions and empyema may occur with any infecting organism but are commoner with *Staph. aureus, Strep. pneumoniae* (and *H. influenzae* in children) and anaerobic organisms.

The clinical features associated with pleural effusion complicating pneumonia depend on the quantity of fluid and whether it is a simple parapneumonic effusion or an empyema. The former often goes unnoticed if small but appears as signs of fluid on the plain chest radiograph. It is rare for a parapneumonic effusion to be so large that it causes additional respiratory embarrassment. The development of an empyema is often accompanied by a slowing of improvement or a worsening of the clinical condition, a return of fever and possibly leukocytosis. The signs of pneumonia become overshadowed by signs of fluid in the pleural space which can be confirmed by ultrasonography or radiology (Fig. 4). The empyema often becomes loculated, which makes management even more difficult.

The differentiation between a benign parapneumonic effusion and an empyema which may become complicated is based on the clinical picture and the characteristics of the pleural fluid (Table 1).

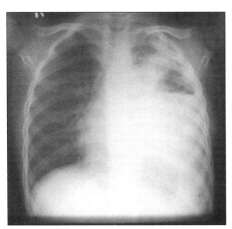

Figure 4
Plain chest radiograph showing an empyema with an air-fluid level in a 9-year-old child with Strep. pneumoniae pneumonia.

Clinical picture and pleural fluid characteristics	Parapneumonic effusion	Empyema
May be coincidental finding	Yes	No
Often associated with persistent or recurrent fever	No	Yes
Clinical and radiological signs of pleural fluid	Yes– usually small	Yes– may be loculated
Cell count > 50 000/μl	Yes	Yes
pH of fluid < 7.2	No	Yes
LDH > 1000 IU/ml	No	Yes
Protein concentration high	Yes	Yes
Responds to treatment of underlying pneumonia	Yes	No
Requires tube or surgical drainage	No	Yes

Table 1
Differentiation between a parapneumonic effusion and an empyema.

Once loculation has developed in an empyema it may take weeks rather than days for the process to resolve, even with appropriate antibiotic therapy and tube drainage. There may be persistent signs of pleural thickening and/or fluid on examination and the chest radiograph remains abnormal. A chest computed tomography (CT) scan often reveals very extensive changes both within the lung and in the pleural space with atelectasis, loculation, fluid and pleural thickening. Surprisingly enough, in most patients these changes can completely reverse with appropriate treatment and with the passage of time.

Differential diagnosis of pneumonia

The clinical presentation of infective pneumonia depends to a large extent on the age and immunological status of the patient and the nature of the organism. Often the diagnosis of pneumonia is very clear clinically or with the aid of simple investigations such as a chest radiograph and blood count. There are circumstances when alternative diagnoses need to be considered.

In the infant

Hyaline membrane disease: occurs in premature infants with typical radiological changes (ground glass appearance).

Meconium aspiration: occurs more often in larger infants with meconium staining of the liquor amnii.

Congenital diaphragmatic hernia: more common on the left side; presence of gut or abdominal viscera in the hemithorax.

Lobar emphysema with atelectasis of another lobe: typical radiological picture of hyperinflation, usually of the upper lobe compressing the lower lobe.

Cystic adenomatoid malformation: may be asymptomatic; typical radiological and CT picture.

Sequestration: typical site and CT picture; may become infected.

In most of these conditions the diagnosis should be obvious from the clinical picture, changes seen on the chest radiograph or CT scan, and the lack of evidence of acute infection. It is particularly important to consider alternative diagnoses in the infant with an infiltrate or atelectasis on the chest radiograph and little or no clinical sign of acute infection.

In the child or adult

Asthma with mucus plugging ('middle lobe syndrome' – may also affect lingula and sometimes other lobes): recurrent respiratory illnesses with symptom-free intervals; good response to anti-asthma medication.

Mucoid impaction syndrome (bronchocentric granulomatosis): recurrent episodes of major bronchial obstruction usually in the left lower lobe, expectoration of bronchial casts, typical histology of casts.

Non-infective interstitial lung disease: non-febrile progressive restrictive lung disease with hypoxia corrected by oxygen inhalation and characteristic changes on lung biopsy.

Non-infective pneumonia: e.g. eosinophilic pneumonia.

Hydatid cyst: characteristic radiological appearance in patients residing in sheep farming areas; may be completely asymptomatic.

Congenital anomalies of lung tissue, airways or mediastinum: bronchogenic cysts and other congenital anomalies have characteristic radiological and CT pictures.

Lymphoma and other malignancies: radiological or CT picture may be typical or there may be evidence of malignancy elsewhere in the body.

Secondary to congenital or valvular heart disease: pulmonary congestion can be mistaken for bronchopneumonia; radiological changes and clinical picture help in diagnosis.

Abdominal pathology: reaction in lung above diaphragm, e.g. pancreatitis, subphrenic abscess.

Most young persons with pneumonia present with a florid picture suggesting infection and lung involvement unless the patient is immunocompromised through disease or through treatment. Alternative diagnoses should always be considered when the clinical or radiological picture is unusual. The misdiagnosis of asthma as pneumonia is very common, especially since many exacerbations of asthma are secondary to upper respiratory tract viral infections so that the patient has signs of infection, abnormal findings on auscultation of the chest and often an abnormal chest radiograph. Malignancy should be suspected in heavy cigarette smokers and in patients with current or previous malignant disease involving other organs.

In the elderly

Chronic obstructive pulmonary disease (COPD): a chronic, generally non-febrile illness with static radiological changes unless complicated by an acute infection, e.g. by pneumonia.

Primary and secondary lung malignancies: radiological or CT picture may be typical or there may be evidence of malignancy elsewhere in the body.

Congestive heart failure: clinical picture, physical signs, cardiomegaly; look for Kerley B lines on the chest radiograph.

Pulmonary embolism (younger adults as well): acute dyspnoea and chest pain, pleural based wedge-shaped lesion; differentiation from pneumonia may require isotope lung scan or angiography.

Pleural diseases: CT scan shows disease to be pleural, not parenchymal, which also distinguishes this problem from an empyema complicating pneumonia.

Pulmonary vascular disease, eosinophilic pneumonia, Wegener's granulomatosis etc: often part of systemic illness; diagnosis is usually made on biopsy.

Simple, uncomplicated pneumonia due to infection does occur in the older patient and it is important to realize that it may take 6 weeks or more for the chest radiograph to return to normal. However, other causes of an abnormal chest radiograph are also common and the possibility of primary or secondary malignant disease must always be considered. Heart failure is also common and it may be difficult to decide whether crepitations at the lung bases are due to fluid overload or to pneumonia in an elderly patient who may not produce florid signs of infection. It may be impossible to decide whether cardiac failure predisposed the patient to infection or whether infection precipitated heart failure. Pulmonary embolism and pulmonary vascular disease may produce radiological changes which are difficult to distinguish from pneumonia, and additional investigations are needed in such patients.

Investigation of pneumonia

The diagnosis of pneumonia can be made on clinical grounds in most patients and, indeed, many are successfully treated each year on an ambulatory basis without any ancillary investigations of any kind. However, in some situations the clinical condition of the patient or an unclear diagnosis makes ancillary investigations desirable. Those available to the clinician include chest radiography and CT scan, microbiological and haematological studies, ultrasonography, studies of pleural fluid, bronchoscopy and lung biopsy. Tests of lung function other than the measurement of arterial blood gases are rarely indicated in the acute phase of an infective pneumonia. Asthma is often misdiagnosed as recurrent pneumonia, especially in children, and bronchial plugging with radiological changes and possible superinfection are also common in this condition. If asthma is suspected, spirometry should be performed before and after the administration of an effective bronchodilator. If the diagnosis is still in doubt, bronchial provocation tests by the inhalation of methacholine or histamine or by physical exercise may be used to document bronchial hyperreactivity. In some patients, especially young children, the only option may be to study the effect of good anti-asthma medication on the course of apparently recurrent pneumonia.

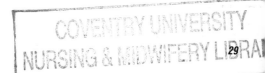

Given that the young healthy adult with classical bacterial pneumonia can probably be safely managed without any ancillary investigations, which investigations are desirable or essential for which patients?

Chest radiograph	All infants and young children and all in whom diagnosis is not certain
	All patients who are seriously ill
	All patients with suspicion of complications of pneumonia
	Desirable in almost all patients after recovery to be sure that nothing has been overlooked
Sputum microscopy and culture	Desirable in all seriously ill patients
	Essential if unusual organism is suspected
	Impossible to obtain from small children except by bronchoscopy, although nasopharyngeal swab may be helpful
	Culture endotracheal tube in intubated patients
Arterial blood gases	Important in all seriously ill patients
	Repeat for monitoring progress
Blood culture	Important in all seriously ill patients before starting antibiotic treatment
Haematological and biochemical investigations	Often helpful in differential diagnosis
	May give an indication of the severity of infection
	Suggestive changes with some infections (adenovirus, *Legionella*)
Serological tests	Rising antibody titre is helpful retrospectively for identifying the organism
	Mainly useful for viral and *Mycoplasma* pneumonia
	Cold agglutinins present in >50% of *Mycoplasma* pneumonia
Ultrasonography	Helpful in identifying pleural fluid and as an aid to pleurocentesis

Chest CT scan	Diagnosis of loculated empyema
	Diagnosis of underlying malignancy
	Diagnosis of other serious pathology
Pleurocentesis, cytology and culture of pleural fluid	All patients with clinical/radiological evidence of a significant pleural effusion
Bronchoscopy	All patients with suspected foreign body aspiration
	All patients with suspected bronchial obstruction
	All patients with suspected congenital anomalies
Bronchoalveolar lavage/ transbronchial biopsy	All patients with severe disease and unknown pathogenesis
	Very important in immunocompromised patients
	All patients with deteriorating condition and unknown pathogen
Open lung biopsy	Patients with persistent or deteriorating pneumonia of uncertain origin and without positive diagnosis by other means
Lung function tests	When asthma is suspected
	For interstitial pneumonia, especially if non-infective in origin

The plain chest radiograph

Almost all patients suspected of having pneumonia should have a plain radiograph of the chest taken as both a postero-anterior and a lateral projection (Fig. 5). This is particularly important in infants and young children in whom the physical signs of pneumonia may be very difficult to elicit reliably. It is also important in those in whom the clinical picture is uncertain, as is often the case in the elderly and in the immunocompromised patient. Homogeneous lobar or segmental shadows are more common than diffuse patchy shadows in bacterial pneumonia and are also seen in over half the patients with atypical pneumonia. In nosocomial infections there are most commonly patchy changes in one or both lower lobes, sometimes with atelectasis. Multiple peripheral discrete fluffy or nodular shadows may suggest a haematogenous origin of the infection. The presence of small amounts of pleural fluid cannot be diagnosed reliably by physical examination and a decubitus lateral chest radiograph (or ultrasonography) is often the best way of detecting this complication of pneumonia. Fluid may be missed on a chest film taken with an infant lying supine on the radiology table, and when in doubt, a suspended, sitting or decubitus lateral film should be taken. The radiological signs of pneumonia may lag behind the clinical course of the disease and it may be necessary to repeat the examination after a day or two (Fig. 6) or if the development of a complication is suspected. Even in patients who have not required extensive investigations and have responded well to treatment,

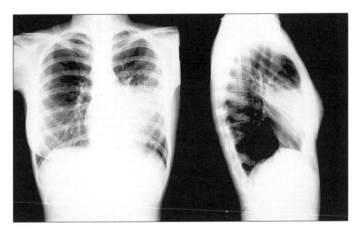

Figure 5
Lobar pneumonia invoving the lingula in a young adult. The lobar location of the infection is best seen on the lateral film.

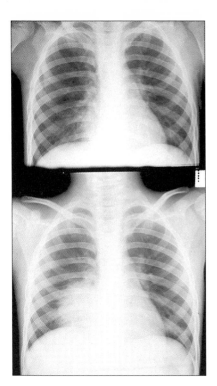

Figure 6
Radiological changes of pneumonia appearing over the course of one day in a 7-year-old-child who presented with cough and fever. The lower film was taken 24 hours after the upper.

a follow-up chest radiograph should be taken after recovery to confirm resolution and to exclude any underlying pathology.

When an infiltrate or cavity is found on the plain chest radiograph, it may be due to a number of processes other than infective pneumonia:

Differential diagnosis of an infiltrate on the plain chest radiograph includes:

- Infective pneumonia of all types – lung volume retained
- Atelectasis – look for decrease in lung volume
- Pleural disease – crosses anatomical lung divisions
- Pulmonary embolism – typically wedge-shaped with pleural base
- Malignancy, including primary and metastatic tumours, lymphomas and blood dyscrasias
- Vasculitis, interstitial non-infective lung disease, lymphangitic spread of malignancy – interstitial pattern
- BOOP – bilateral multiple infiltrates changing with time
- Eosinophilic pneumonia – peripheral infiltrates with central sparing
- Congenital anomalies of lung, airways, mediastinal tissues – typical location of lesion

Differential diagnosis of a cavity on the plain chest radiograph includes:

- Pneumatocele secondary to necrotizing pneumonia. This usually appears during the course of otherwise typical clinical and radiological pneumonia. Cysts are usually thin-walled and multiple, and may become fluid-filled. A previous normal chest radiograph is helpful in distinguishing this lesion from other cystic lesions. Fungi may infect an existing cyst or the fungus may be the primary infecting agent. In typical cases a fungus ball can be seen surrounded by a clear halo within the cyst.
- Infection in a pre-existing single or multiple cystic lesion of the lung. This may be difficult to distinguish from pneumatocele unless there is a previous chest radiograph showing the lesion. Congenital cysts and congenital cystic adenomatoid malformations may become infected.
- Lung abscess due to complicated pneumonia, aspiration of foreign material or infected pulmonary embolism. The cyst wall is usually thick and the surrounding lung tissue relatively healthy. The clue lies in the clinical circumstances and the radiological picture.
- Necrosis of lung tissue within a malignant lesion or within a pulmonary infarction. The clinical picture is not normally one of acute infection and there should be other clues to the correct diagnosis.

Ultrasonography

Ultrasonography of the thorax is primarily used to confirm the clinical impression of the presence of pleural fluid and as a guide to thoracentesis. The presence of loculations in an empyema may also be demonstrated in some patients. Ultrasonography is non-invasive and does not involve irradiation and is therefore preferable to radiological studies so long as it provides the required information. Unfortunately, even in expert hands ultrasonography may be quite unreliable and the patient will also require a CT scan.

Chest CT scan

There is no doubt that far too many CT scans of the chest are performed in patients with uncomplicated pneumonia. On the other hand, a CT scan can be very helpful when the differential diagnosis is complicated and is the only reliable way of evaluating the extent and location of a loculated empyema (Fig. 7). The correct placement of a pleural drainage tube may only be possible under CT control. The radiological image obtained by a CT scan in the patient with pneumonia is often much more florid than that on the plain radiograph and it is important to realize that quite extensive abnormalities seen on the CT scan can clear completely with time. A CT scan is more reliable than a plain radiograph in detecting pathology underlying pneumonia, such as a bronchial carcinoma, and should always be requested when there is suspicion of serious underlying pathology (Fig. 8). Foreign body aspiration should be diagnosed by bronchoscopy, as the CT scan is often unreliable in such cases.

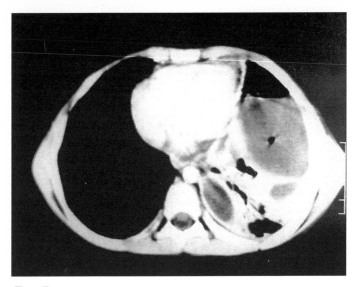

Figure 7
Chest CT scan showing extensive loculated empyema with many septae not visible on the plain chest radiograph.

Laboratory investigations

Blood cultures

These are easy to perform and very informative when positive. If possible, obtain before starting antibiotic therapy; otherwise, obtain at the end of a dosage interval.

1. Disinfect skin with 70% alcohol and then povidone-iodine, and allow to take effect for at least 1 min. It is important to disinfect the palpating finger also. Do not use venous cannulae or indwelling catheters.
2. Take a 10-ml sample (2 ml for children) and divide it between two prewarmed bottles for aerobic and anaerobic culture. Disinfect the stoppers of the bottles before injecting the blood.
3. If immediate transport to the laboratory is not possible, incubate the bottles at 37°C.

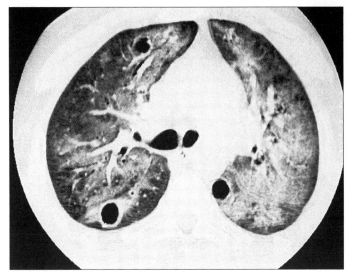

Figure 8
Chest CT scan in a patient with AIDS and an interstitial pneumonia due to Pneumocystis carinii infection. There are widespread interstitial changes and large cystic spaces with honeycombing are also present. This picture is from the patient whose plain chest radiograph is shown in Fig.3.

Pleural fluid

This should always be sampled when present.

After disinfection of the skin as above, obtain the sample by percutaneous needle aspiration. About 5 ml should be sent for microscopy and culture, but >10 ml if mycobacteria or fungi are suspected. Samples could also be sent for protein content, sugar, pH, lactate dehydrogenase, cytology (inflammatory cell type and malignant cells), microscopy and culture for acid-fast bacilli.

Sputum

This is often not available during the early stages of pneumonia. However, if available it should be expectorated by a deep cough (sometimes aided by the physiotherapist) into a sterile container. Sputum should be examined by Gram stain which is useful if large numbers of bacteria, e.g. pneumococci or staphylococci, are seen and confirms the sample is from the lower respiratory tract (Figs 9–12).

1. Using a sterile loop, smear the material evenly onto a clean glass slide.

2. Allow to air-dry completely.

3. Heat or alcohol fix the preparation. Heat fixation: pass the slide with the coated side upwards several times through a yellow flame. Alcohol fixation: flood the slide with methanol for 3 min and then pour off.

4. Flood the slide with crystal violet or carbo-gentian violet for 1 min and then pour off.

5. Flood with Gram's iodine for 1 min and then pour off.

6. Decolorize with ethanol/acetone (96% ethanol with 3% acetone) until any colour is released.

7. Rinse with water.

8. Counterstain with safranin or carbol-fuchsin for 15–30 s.

9. Rinse with water and blot with absorbent paper.

10. Examine under a microscope without a coverslip at x 1000 magnification: x 10 eyepiece and x 100 oil-immersion lens. Elevate the condenser and open the diaphragm completely.

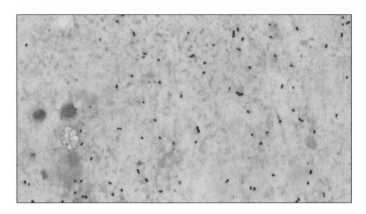

Figure 9
Strep. pneumoniae in a sputum sample.

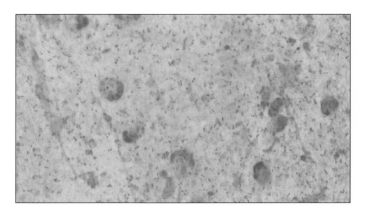

Figure 10
P. aeruginosa in a sputum sample.

11. Gram-positive bacteria will appear dark blue or purple, while Gram-negative bacteria will stain light or deep red.

12. Less than 10 squamous cells per high-power field and more than 25 neutrophils per high-power field make lung infection likely.

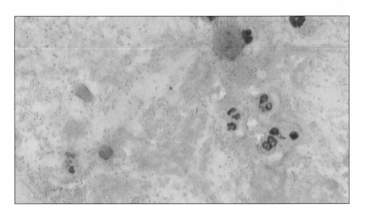

Figure 11
Klebsiella pneumoniae in a sputum sample.

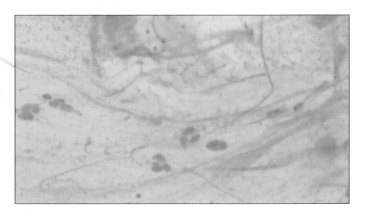

Figure 12
H. influenzae in a sputum sample.

Sputum should be transported promptly to the laboratory for culture (washing or homogenization and dilution may overcome contamination by upper respiratory tract commensals). Prior antibiotics frequently suppress bacterial growth, especially of *Strep. pneumoniae* and *H. influenzae*. A nasopharyngeal swab may be helpful in children who do not produce sputum.

Polysaccharide capsular antigen of pneumococci can be detected in sputum, pleural fluid, urine or blood by countercurrent immunoelectrophoresis. This increases diagnostic yield but is not available in most laboratories; it is also best suited to batch testing, and so is not ideal for emergency specimens.

Haematology

A raised white cell count is usual in bacterial pneumonia, but in atypical (except *Legionella*) or viral pneumonia it is usually normal.

Biochemistry

Mildly abnormal liver function tests are quite common in pneumonia. Raised blood urea, hypocalcaemia, hypoalbuminaemia and hyponatraemia all occur in severe pneumonia, the latter most commonly with *Legionella* infection.

Serology

Because culture techniques are unavailable or difficult, viral and atypical pneumonias can be diagnosed retrospectively by a four-fold or greater rise in specific antibody titre in acute and convalescent serum. Acute serum should be sent at presentation and convalescent serum about 14 days later. Direct fluorescent antibody staining of respiratory secretions or lavage material can make the diagnosis of viral and atypical pneumonias immediately; however, these tests may not be available in routine laboratories. Serum can be sent for cold agglutinins, which are positive in over half of *Mycoplasma* pneumonias.

Invasive procedures

These should be considered to obtain uncontaminated secretions, and/or tissue for culture and histology, in all seriously ill patients, particularly when there is doubt about diagnosis. The following investigations may be performed depending on the clinical circumstances and the site and extent of the pulmonary lesion: transtracheal aspiration, bronchoscopic aspiration and protected brush catheter, bronchoalveolar lavage, trans-bronchial biopsy, percutaneous fine-needle aspiration, percu-taneous (CT-guided) needle biopsy, open lung biopsy. In all these investigations there must be very close liaison between the clinician and microbiologist.

Management of pneumonia and its complications in hospital

The objective of correct management of established pneumonia is to support the vital bodily functions of the patient and to find the best method of helping the natural defences of the patient to overcome the infection. This depends upon the nature of the infecting organisms and the antimicrobial therapy available. Since the natural course of the disease and the commonest infecting organism vary according to the type of patient, different approaches to management are needed for the different groups of patients. At each stage the physician must make certain important decisions and be prepared to revise them in the light of the response of the patient. These questions include:

- Whether the patient should be hospitalized
- Whether there are confounding factors increasing the danger to the patient
- How severe the disease is at the present time
- What, if any, investigations are needed
- What is the most likely organism causing the pneumonia
- What is the most appropriate treatment
- How the patient has responded to treatment received so far
- Whether treatment should be changed
- Whether further investigations are needed to detect complications
- Whether the diagnosis of infective pneumonia is correct
- Whether there is underlying pathology

In the past the commonest bacteria causing pneumonia acquired in the community were sensitive to penicillin or its analogues and this also applied to pneumococci, which remained very susceptible, with a mean inhibitory concentration (MIC) for benzylpenicillin of less than 0.6 mg/l. More recently the problem of penicillin-resistant pneumococci has arisen; this was first noted in Australia. There were then occasional isolates reported from elsewhere, but the majority had low-level resistance to penicillin, with MICs between 0.1 and 1 mg/l. However, by 1978 strains with high-level resistance to penicillin (MIC ≥ 2 mg/l), often with associated resistance to several other classes of antibiotic, had been isolated, first in South Africa and subsequently elsewhere. In Spain, particularly, invasive disease due to multiresistant pneumococci has become a common clinical problem.

Penicillin resistance arises by evolution of penicillin-resistant forms of the penicillin-binding proteins. Whether penicillin resistance should influence treatment of pneumococcal infections depends on the degree of resistance and the site of infection. Meningitis caused by pneumococci with any degree of penicillin insensitivity is associated with a poor response and a high mortality even with high-dose penicillin therapy. However, for pneumonia it is only high-level resistance which affects response to treatment. At the moment penicillin-resistant strains, particularly of the high-level variety, are very infrequent in the UK, and the guidelines for therapy need not yet be adjusted. Resistance to penicillin is linked to that for other antibiotics, and various patterns of resistance have been described – the most resistant isolates being resistant to all beta-lactam antibiotics, chloramphenicol, erythromycin, tetracycline, clindamycin and rifampicin. Vancomycin might be considered for first-line therapy should these strains become more prevalent in the UK, or for a patient with pneumonia returning from a holiday in Spain.

General management of pneumonia in specific groups of patients

The following are general recommendations for the management of pneumonia in patients who require hospitalization. The management of pneumonia in a communal setting without hospitalization is considered in the next chapter. The recommended choices of antibiotics for the different types of patient are given in the chapter starting on page 59 and the recommended doses of the drugs in Appendix B on page 69.

Management of pneumonia in the newborn and young infant

Pneumonia in the newborn nursery is not particularly common but can be rapidly fatal if due to Group B streptococcal infection. In most cases it is wise to begin treatment with a wide-spectrum combination such as ampicillin and gentamicin, with all due care for the correct dose, which is lower during the first week of life because of the relatively poor renal function in the immediate newborn period. Infections may also be due to *Chlamydia,* although this is rarely a problem before the age of 2–3 weeks. The premature infant is susceptible to a variety of nosocomial infections and the differentiation between pneumonia and sepsis is often academic, since all such infants (and all other seriously ill infants in the first 4 weeks of life) require a full sepsis investigation, including a lumbar puncture. Pneumonia in older infants is often due to *H. influenzae,* which requires a combination of ampicillin and a beta-lactamase inhibitor (Augmentin), trimethoprim/sulphamethoxazole, or a second/third-generation cephalosporin.

Hospitalization	Definitely indicated, high-risk patient
	Can be difficult to diagnose and manage
	Invariably requires parenteral therapy
	Can be rapidly fatal if mismanaged
Evaluation of severity by	General alertness, willingness to take feeds
	Oxygen requirements, presence of apnoeic spells
	Tachypnoea, tachycardia
Initial investigations needed	Chest radiograph
	Pulse oximetry and/or arterial blood gas evaluation
	Full blood picture
	Thrombocyte count
	Blood culture
	Lumbar puncture to exclude meningitis – almost always needed
	Serum biochemistry
Likeliest organisms	Group B streptococci
	Staphylococci
	E. coli, other enterobacteriacae
	Chlamydia (over 2–3 weeks)
	H. influenzae (older infants)
	Viruses
General management	Tube feeding if too distressed to suck well
	Intravenous feeding if very sick
	Adequate hydration, good urine output
	Added oxygen to maintain saturation >93%
Initial empirical antibiotic therapy	See page 59. Subsequent treatment depends upon the response and results of cultures.
Evaluating the response	General alertness, feeding
	Pulse oximeter saturation
	Oxygen requirements, apnoeic spells
	Thrombocyte count
	Follow-up chest radiograph

cont'd

Alternative treatment/aetiology if response is poor	Consider changing antibiotic
	Consider RSV infection, especially if infant is wheezy
	Consider using ribavirin if: (a) RSV is identified in secretions; (b) infant is severely ill; and (c) other disease present e.g. congenital heart disease
	Consider bronchopulmonary dysplasia (BPD) in the premature infant
Complications to consider	Pneumatoceles
	Pneumothorax
	Pneumomediastinum
	Empyema (rare)
Differential diagnoses to consider	Hyaline membrane disease
	Meconium aspiration
	Heart failure
	Congenital anomalies

Management of pneumonia in the older child or adult

The morbidity and even mortality of community-acquired pneumonia is significant in adults, especially in those with negative prognostic features such as advanced age or pre-existing illness. Since several studies have shown that it is usually impossible to identify pathogens on the basis of clinical features and cultures of blood and secretions take 24 h to yield results, while serological diagnosis in atypical pneumonia is retrospective, initiation of treatment is usually empirical. A combination of a beta-lactam antibiotic (e.g. benzylpenicillin, ampicillin, amoxicillin, amoxicillin/clavulanate [Augmentin], or cefuroxime) and a macrolide (e.g. erythromycin) is recommended for seriously ill patients. The macrolide will deal with the atypical infections, e.g. *Mycoplasma, Legionella* and *Chlamydia*, and the beta-lactam with other likely pathogens. Amoxicillin given in combination with the beta-lactamase inhibitor clavulanate (Augmentin) might be the first choice beta-lactam antibiotic. Cefuroxime might be an alternative choice because it is not broken down by the beta-lactamase enzymes of *H. influenzae* and *Moraxella catarrhalis*.

When pneumonia occurs following influenza infection, *Staph. aureus* should be considered and flucloxacillin included in the antibiotic regimen. The mortality of community- acquired pneumonia serious enough to require hospitalization remains up to 5%, despite the use of potent antibiotics and intensive care. This failure of treatment is sometime due to processes independent of the initial infecting organism, e.g. adult respiratory distress syndrome or other organ failure, rather than continued infection or suboptimal management.

Hospitalization	Depends on home circumstances
	Depends on severity of pneumonia
	If patient has two out of three adverse features – tachypnoea, hypotension, renal failure – mortality is increased by 20 times
	Most small children require parenteral therapy initially
	For ambulatory management see next chapter
Evaluation of severity by	Temperature, tachypnoea, blood pressure
	Presence of central cyanosis
	Confusion or drowsiness
	Extent of clinical or radiological disease
Initial investigations needed	Chest radiograph
	Full blood picture and serum biochemistry
	Pulse oximetry saturation (arterial blood gases if very sick)
	Sputum, if available, for microscopy and culture
	Blood culture
	Serology for *Mycoplasma, Legionella* and respiratory viruses
Likeliest organisms	*Streptococcus pneumoniae*
	Mycoplasma pneumoniae
	H. influenzae
	Respiratory viruses
	Legionella, Chlamydia, and *Staphylococcus* are much less common

cont'd

General management	Bed rest
	Encourage fluids
	No smoking
	Oxygen to maintain saturation >93%
	Analgesics for pleural pain
	Paracetamol to reduce fever
Initial empirical antibiotic therapy	See page 60. Subsequent treatment depends upon the response and results of cultures.
Evaluating the response	Fever
	Physical signs
	Blood picture
	Repeat chest radiograph
Alternative treatment aetiology if response is poor	Consider changing the antibiotic
	Viral infection
	Unusual pathogen, e.g. *Legionella*
	Antibiotic resistance
	Consider host defence problem
	Consider coincidental non-pulmonary disease
	Patient not getting antibiotic for some technical reason
Further investigations if patient not improving	Ultrasonography, CT scan to assess pathology
	Pleurocentesis if fluid present
	Serology for viruses, *Legionella* etc.
	Invasive diagnostic procedures, bronchoscopy, bronchoalveolar lavage (BAL), biopsy
	Immunological investigations
Complications to consider	Respiratory failure if patient cannot maintain adequate blood gases
	Empyema
	Lung abscess
	Septic emboli, e.g. arthritis, endocarditis

cont'd

	Adult respiratory distress syndrome
	Drug fever
Differential diagnoses to consider	Malignant disease of lung or pleura
	Interstitial non-infective lung disease
	Eosinophilic pneumonia
	Bronchiolitis obliterans/cryptogenic organizing pneumonia (BOOP/COP)
	Heart failure
	Congenital anomalies, e.g. sequestration

Management of pneumonia in the elderly or debilitated

Hospitalization	Indicated unless home circumstances are ideal or patient is not seriously ill
Possible confounding factors increasing the danger	COPD
	Ischaemic heart disease
	Hypertension
	Heart failure
	Diabetes
	Renal failure
	Reduced immune response to infection
Difference in the management compared with the younger patient	Temperature – not always much elevated
	Confusion or reduced well-being may be the only symptom
	ECG should always be included in initial investigations
	H. influenzae and other Gram-negative bacilli are more common
	Mycoplasma infection is less common
	Other coexistent pathology is likely to require treatment

cont'd

	Pulmonary embolism may present a similar clinical picture
	Always remember the possibility of tuberculosis
Initial empirical antibiotic therapy	See page 59. Subsequent treatment depends upon the response and results of cultures.
Evaluating the response	Fever – not very helpful
	Physical signs – not very helpful
	General well-being, level of confusion
	Repeat chest radiograph – essential

Management of nosocomial pneumonia

- Consider pathogenesis as this may alter management or choice of antibiotic
- Prior COPD – pathogen may be *H. influenzae* or *Strep. pneumoniae*
- Prior antibiotic therapy – antibiotic-resistant Gram-negative bacilli may have colonized the nasopharynx and been aspirated
- Gastro-oesophageal aspiration – anaerobes may be involved
- Ventilator, nebulizer or suction equipment may be the source of infection
- Reduced cough, e.g. due to pain or drugs, hinders clearance of secretions
- Blood spread of infection from distant focus, e.g. abdominal sepsis giving multiple discrete or fluffy shadows on chest radiograph – treat primary site
- Condition causing hospital admission may complicate the picture, e.g. cerebrovascular accident
- Anaerobic infection is more frequent
- If blood and sputum cultures and serology are unhelpful, invasive techniques may be required to obtain lower respiratory tract secretions
- Initial empirical antibiotic therapy – see pages 61–2. Subsequent treatment depends upon the response and results of cultures.

Management of pneumonia in the immunocompromised patient

Hospitalization	Definitely indicated, high-risk patient
	Can be difficult to diagnose and manage
	Invariably requires parenteral therapy
Possible confounding factors increasing the danger	Susceptibility to unusual organisms
	Very poor host defences
	Coincident disease, e.g. malignancy, transplant rejection
	Graft versus host disease in transplant recipient
	May be receiving immunosuppressant drugs
Evaluation of severity by	Temperature – not always much elevated
	Inspired oxygen requirements, blood gases
	Tachypnoea, blood pressure
	Chest radiograph
Initial investigations needed	Chest radiograph
	CT scan often helps delineate disease and assess severity
	Full blood picture and serum biochemistry
	Sputum, blood and pleural fluid for microscopy and culture
	Pulse oximeter saturation or blood gases
	Bronchoscopy with bronchoalveolar lavage and transbronchial biopsy
	Serology for HIV, respiratory viruses, *Mycoplasma, Legionella, Aspergillus* etc.
Likeliest organisms	If neutrophils are reduced – bacteria and fungi
	If immunoglobulin deficient – bacteria
	If T-lymphocyte problem – viruses, especially herpes group, CMV, mycobacteria and *Pneumocystis carinii*
Initial empirical antibiotic therapy	See page 62. Subsequent treatment depends upon the response and results of cultures.

cont'd

Evaluating the response	Fever, physical signs
	Repeat chest radiograph
	Inspired oxygen requirements
Alternative treatment/aetiology if response is poor	Consider changing antibiotic
	Consider ganciclovir for CMV infection
	Consider adding corticosteroids in *Pneumocystis carinii* infection
Further investigations if patient not improving	Bronchoscopy/BAL, transbronchial biopsy if not already performed
	Open lung biopsy if bronchoscopic investigations inconclusive
Differential diagnoses to consider	Malignancy, lymphoma, leukaemia
	Pulmonary oedema, haemorrhage, infarction
	Radiation pneumonitis
	Drug-induced pneumonitis (bulsuphan, cyclophosphamide, methotrexate)
	BOOP/COP
	Transplant rejection, graft versus host disease
	Alveolar proteinosis

Management of pulmonary tuberculosis

Hospitalization	Hospital admission and isolation are not required
	Give general advice, e.g. avoidance of droplet spread by cough
	Screen direct contacts
	Patients are non-infectious 2 weeks after commencing effective treatment
Evaluation of severity by	Weight loss, general well-being
	Physical signs of lung disease
	Chest radiograph

cont'd

	Number of organisms in sputum smear; only smear positive patients are infectious
Initial investigations needed	Chest radiograph
	Sputum for smear and culture – a new, rapid test, the BACTEC radiometric system, detects mycobacteria in about 2 weeks and gives antibiotic sensitivities in 4 weeks
	Full blood picture and serum biochemistry
	Aspiration of pleural fluid (if present) and pleural biopsy – bacteria are sparse, lymphocytes predominate and high-protein-content, pleural granulomas
Initial empirical antibiotic therapy	See page 65. Subsequent treatment depends upon the response and results of cultures
Evaluating the response	Temperature
	Chest radiograph
	Loss of systemic symptoms, e.g. night sweats
	Weight gain
	Sputum smear (reduction in number of bacilli) and culture (no growth, dead bacilli seen on sputum smear will continue to be produced for some weeks)

Possible toxic effect of drugs used to treat tuberculosis

Isoniazid: hepatotoxicity occurs in 1–2% of patients; peripheral neuropathy due to pyridoxine deficiency occurs in up to 2% of patients on high doses not given pyridoxine prophylactically.

Rifampicin: colours secretions, e.g. urine and tears, red which may stain (must warn contact lens wearers); liver enzyme induction increases metabolism and reduces effectiveness of many drugs, e.g. corticosteroids, contraceptive pill, anticonvulsants; hepatotoxicity; transient blood dyscrasias; more severe immune reactions occur, especially with intermittent use, which may give a "flu-like" syndrome.

Pyrazinamide: arthralgia; gout; hepatotoxicity.

Ethambutol: retrobulbar neuritis – this is less common at 15 mg/kg dosage, but all patients given ethambutol must stop taking drug immediately if there is any loss of visual acuity; most of the drug is excreted unchanged in the urine, so it should not be given, if possible, to patients with impaired renal function.

Management of pneumonia in the community

The primary care physician, as well as deciding on what treatment to prescribe, must decide which patients are referred to hospital. Almost all babies and young children with pneumonia will be referred to hospital, but most adults with community-acquired pneumonia will be managed at home. One must bear in mind that there remains a significant mortality from community-acquired pneumonia, particularly when associated with recognized negative prognostic features (see below). This chapter describes management of the older child and adult patient with pneumonia at home. For determination of whether the patient has pneumonia, see Table 2.

	Pneumonia	Heart failure	Asthma	Chronic bronchitis
Fever	+++	– – –	– – –	+ –
Cough and sputum	++	– – –	+	+++
Breathlessness	++	++	+++	+
Malaise, confusion	++	+	– – –	– – –
Bronchial breathing	+++	– – –	– – –	– – –
Localized crepitations	++	++	+ –	++
Generalized wheezing	– – –	+	+++	++
Peripheral oedema	– – –	+++	– – –	– – –

Table 2
Has the patient got pneumonia?

The following features would favour immediate referral to hospital:

- Poor home circumstances
- Confusion
- Age >60 years
- Pre-existing respiratory medical condition, e.g. COPD, asthma, emphysema
- Pre-existing non-respiratory medical condition, e.g. diabetes, heart failure, renal failure
- Respiratory rate >30/min (adult)
- Hypotension, diastolic BP < 60 mmHg (adult)
- Cyanosis
- Extremes of temperature, either high (>40°C) or low (< 35°C)
- Evidence on auscultation of widespread involvement
- Evidence of pleural fluid on examination
- Pneumonia following a flu-like illness suggests possibility of staphylococcal infection
- Recent foreign travel

In most cases no investigations will be performed but the following might occasionally be considered:

- Domiciliary chest radiograph if available. Multilobe involvement suggests a worse prognosis. Coexistent disease, e.g. heart failure or carcinoma, may be present
- Full blood picture. White cell count < 4000/mm^3 or >30 000/mm^3 suggests a worse prognosis. With pneumococcal or *Haemophilus* pneumonia, the white cell count is usually >15 000/mm^3. With viral or atypical pneumonia, the white cell count is often near normal
- Urea and electrolytes. Blood urea >7 mmol/l suggests a worse prognosis. Hyponatraemia occurs in severe pneumonia, most commonly with *Legionella*
- Sputum for microscopy and culture is rarely useful

The following general advice should be given to the patient and his or her family:

- Rest in bed
- Encourage fluid intake
- Do not smoke
- Take aspirin or paracetamol to control temperature
- Contact the doctor if the condition worsens

The following oral antibiotics are appropriate for treatment:

- Amoxicillin or ampicillin is the treatment of choice in almost all circumstances for the ambulatory management of pneumonia unless the patient is allergic to penicillin, there is a *Mycoplasma* epidemic in the community, or beta-lactamase-producing *H. influenzae* is suspected
- Erythromycin is the initial treatment of choice if the patient is allergic to penicillin or there is a *Mycoplasma* epidemic in the community, but remember that *H. influenzae* is not sensitive to erythromycin
- Augmentin (clavulanic acid plus amoxicillin) is preferred if the beta-lactamase-producing *H. influenzae* is suspected
- If the patient has not responded to ampicillin or amoxicillin after 72 h, change to erythromycin
- If the patient is intolerant of erythromycin, change to clarithromycin

The following features would suggest that a patient being managed at home should be transferred to hospital:

- Increasing respiratory rate
- Increasing tachycardia
- Falling blood pressure
- Onset of confusion
- Development of cyanosis
- Increased signs on auscultation
- Development of signs of pleural effusion
- Failure of temperature to settle

Antibiotics used for the management of pneumonia in hospital

Antibiotics affect both host and micro-organism, and can have both beneficial and adverse effects. To choose an antibiotic, one should know the infecting organism, or, failing this, the organisms that are commonly implicated in a particular clinical presentation. It is also critical to know the antibiotic sensitivity of the strains likely to be encountered. Successful outcome of treatment will depend upon the type of infection, the virulence and antibiotic sensitivity of the pathogen, the status of the host defences, the presence or absence of pre-existing disease of the lung, the existence or not of other illness, and the choice of antibiotic therapy. The following considers the antibiotic choices available for the treatment of particular types of pneumonia and pneumonia in particular patient groups. The recommended doses of the various drugs are given in Appendix B on page 69. For most uncomplicated bacterial pneumonias the duration of antibiotic therapy should be about 7–10 days, but the duration of treatment will vary from case to case depending upon the infecting agent and the response of the patient.

Pneumonia in the newborn and infant

In the otherwise healthy full-term newborn infant during the first month of life:

- IV ampicillin plus IV gentamicin (or amikacin, tobramycin)

Notes: (1) Lower doses used in the first 2 weeks of life.
(2) Dosage of aminoglycosides is dependent on patient size and renal function and serum levels should be monitored.

If the pathogen is suspected to be a Group B *Streptococcus:*

- IV penicillin G plus IV gentamicin (or amikacin, tobramycin)

Notes: (1) Lower doses used in the first 2 weeks of life.
(2) Dosage of aminoglycosides is dependent on patient size and renal function and serum levels should be monitored.

In the premature infant and for nosocomial infections in the nursery:

- IV vancomycin (or teicoplanin) plus IV cefotaxime (or ceftriaxone)

Note: (1) Lower doses used in first two weeks of life.

Older infants (usually >2–3 weeks) with signs of *Chlamydia* infection:

- IV erythromycin

Community-acquired pneumonia in the older child and adult

- IV amoxicillin/clavulanate plus oral or IV erythromycin
- IV cefuroxime plus oral or IV erythromycin

Notes: (1) Intravenous erythromycin is very irritant to veins – either administer in sodium chloride 0.9% or use long line.
(2) If penicillin allergic, use cephalosporin as above with caution (possibility of cross-sensitivity) or IV erythromycin alone.

Empyema

- IV clindamycin plus IV gentamicin (or amikacin, tobramycin)

Alternative:

- IV imipenem plus IV gentamicin (or amikacin, tobramycin)

Note: (1) Dosage of aminoglycosides is dependent on patient size and renal function and serum levels should be monitored.

Lung abscess

- IV piperacillin (or ticarcillin) plus IV or rectal metronidazole

Alternative:

- IV imipenem plus IV gentamicin (or amikacin, tobramycin)

Note: (1) Dosage of aminoglycosides is dependent on patient size and renal function and serum levels should be monitored.

Nosocomial pneumonia (in the general wards)

- IV amoxicillin/clavulanate plus IV gentamicin
- IV piperacillin (or ticarcillin) plus IV gentamicin (or amikacin, tobramycin)

Alternative:

- Ceftriaxone (or IV cefotaxime) plus IV gentamicin (or amikacin, tobramycin)

Note: (1) Dosage of aminoglycosides is dependent on patient size and renal function and serum levels should be monitored.

Nosocomial pneumonia (in ICU)

- IV ceftazidime plus IV gentamicin (or amikacin, tobramycin)

Alternatives:

- IV imipenem plus gentamicin (or amikacin, tobramycin)
- IV ciprofloxacin plus IV gentamicin (or amikacin, tobramycin)

- IV tazocin plus IV gentamicin (or amikacin, tobramycin)

Notes: (1) Dosage of aminoglycosides is dependent on patient size and renal function and serum levels should be monitored. (2) Vancomycin (or teicoplanin) can be added for extra streptococcal and staphylococcal cover. (3) Local experience of P. aeruginosa gentamicin resistance may make amikacin the first-choice aminoglycoside.

Aspiration pneumonia

- Ceftriaxone (or IV cefotaxime) plus IV or rectal metronidazole

Alternative :

- IV imipenem plus IV gentamicin (or amikacin, tobramycin)

Notes: (1) Dosage of aminoglycosides is dependent on patient size and renal function and serum levels should be monitored. (2) Infection secondary to foreign body aspiration in a small child is most commonly due to H. influenzae, and cefuroxime should be used.

Pneumonia in the immunocompromised

- IV imipenem plus gentamicin (or amikacin, tobramycin)

Alternatives:

- IV ceftazidime plus IV gentamicin (or amikacin, tobramycin)
- IV ciprofloxacin plus IV gentamicin (or amikacin, tobramycin)
- IV tazocin plus IV gentamicin (or amikacin, tobramycin)

Notes: (1) Dosage of aminoglycosides is dependent on patient size and renal function and serum levels should be monitored. (2) Vancomycin (or teicoplanin) can be added for extra streptococcal and staphylococcal cover. (3) Local experience of P. aeruginosa gentamicin resistance may make amikacin the first-choice aminoglycoside. (4) An abrupt onset with localized shadowing makes bacterial pneumonia most likely.

Aspergillus pneumonia

- IV amphotericin B (or AmBisome – liposome encapsulated amphotericin)

Notes: (1) Hypokalaemia and hypomagnesaemia occur and may need supplements. (2) Addition of IV sodium chloride reduces frequency of nephrotoxicity. (3) Monitor renal function; if it deteriorates, stop amphotericin until it stabilizes and then recommence on an every-other-day schedule. (4) 1 000 units of heparin in the infusion reduces the frequency of thrombophlebitis. (5) IV flucytosine may be used in combination with amphotericin, either because of synergy between the two compounds in a sick patient or to allow a reduction in the amphotericin dosage if there are toxicity problems.

Cryptococcus pneumonia and *Candida* pneumonia

- IV amphotericin B (or AmBisome – liposome encapsulated amphotericin)

Notes: (1) Hypokalaemia and hypomagnesaemia occur and may need supplements. (2) Addition of IV sodium chloride reduces frequency of nephrotoxicity. (3) Monitor renal function; if it deteriorates, stop amphotericin until it stabilizes and then recommence on an every-other-day schedule. (4) 1 000 units of heparin in the infusion reduces the frequency of thrombophlebitis. (5) IV flucytosine may be used in combination with amphotericin, either because of synergy between the two compounds in a sick patient or to allow a reduction in the amphotericin dosage if there are toxicity problems. (6)Therapy can be changed to oral fluconazole as the patient's condition improves.

Cytomegalovirus pneumonia

- IV ganciclovir

Alternative:

- IV foscarnet

Notes: (1) Administration of CMV immunoglobulin may be beneficial. (2) High rate of adverse reactions to foscarnet, so only use in life-threatening infections. (3) Monitor renal function and serum calcium during foscarnet therapy.

Herpes virus pneumonia (Herpes simplex and varicella-zoster)

- IV acyclovir

Nocardia pneumonia

- Oral co-trimoxazole

Alternative:

- Oral minocycline

Pneumocystis pneumonia

- Oral or IV co-trimoxazole

Alternatives:

- IV or nebulized pentamidine isethionate
- Trimethoprim plus dapsone

Psittacosis

- Oral tetracycline

Alternatives:

- Oral doxycycline
- Oral erythromycin

Q fever

•	Oral tetracycline

Alternatives:

•	Oral doxycycline
•	Oral co-trimoxazole

Tuberculosis

•	A combination of oral isoniazid, oral rifampicin and oral pyrazinamide for 2 months, and then isoniazid and rifampicin at the same dosage alone for a further 4 months

Notes: (1) Ethambutol should be added to the initial regimen for the first 2 months if antibiotic resistance is suspected.

Appendix A:
Micro-organisms causing pneumonia

This list is not meant to be exhaustive but to cover the commoner species:

Organism	Description of microscopic examination where applicable
Bacterial pneumonia – community-acquired	
Common	
Streptococcus pneumoniae	Gram-positive diplococci
*Mycoplasma pneumoniae**	
Haemophilus influenzae	Gram-negative bacilli or cocco-bacilli
*Chlamydia pneumoniae**	
*Legionella pneumophila**	
Uncommon	
Klebsiella pneumoniae	Gram-negative bacilli
Staphylococcus aureus	Gram-positive cocci often in clusters

Moraxella catarrhalis	Gram-negative bacilli or cocco-bacilli
*Chlamydia psittaci**	
*Coxiella burnetti**	
Neisseria meningitidis	Intra/extra-leukocytic Gram-negative diplococci
Gram-negative bacilli	See below
Viral pneumonia*	
Influenza A and B	
Respiratory syncytial virus	
Adenovirus	
Parainfluenza virus	
Herpes viruses	
Cytomegalovirus	
Hospital-acquired pneumonia	
Pseudomonas aeruginosa	Gram-negative bacilli
Staphylococcus aureus	Gram-positive cocci
Klebsiella spp.	Gram-negative bacilli
Enterobacter spp.	Gram-negative bacilli
Escherichia coli	Gram-negative bacilli
Streptococcus spp.	Gram-positive cocci
Serratia marcescens	Gram-negative bacilli
Proteus spp.	Gram-negative bacilli
Acinetobacter spp.	Gram-negative bacilli
Citrobacter spp.	Gram-negative bacilli
Anaerobes	

Fungal pneumonia	
Aspergillus fumigatus	Septate branching hyphae in smear or tissue
Aspergillus spp.	Septate branching hyphae in smear or tissue
Cryptococcus neoformans	Encapsulated yeast cells in india ink
Candida albicans	Budding cells, sometimes with pseudo-hyphae
Coccidioides immitis	Spherules with endospores
Blastomyces dermatiditis	Yeast cells in wet mounts or tissue
Histoplasma capsulatum	Intracellular yeast cells
Others	
Mycobacterium tuberculosis	Acid-fast bacilli
Environmental mycobacteria, e.g. *Mycobacterium avium-intracellulare*	Acid-fast bacilli
Pneumocystis carinii	Methanamine silver staining of cysts

* Organisms not seen by routine light microscopy.

Appendix B:
Recommended drug doses

Note: *The doses recommended in this book have been taken from the British National Formulary unless no appropriate dose was described, in which case other sources were used. Every care has been taken to ensure accuracy but the reader must verify the doses he or she prescribes and the authors cannot accept responsibility for any errors resulting from failure to administer the correct dose.*

Acyclovir Antiviral agent used to treat herpes infections.

	<2 years	Child	Adult
Oral/24 h	500–1000 mg	1000–3200 mg	1000–4000mg
IV/24 h	750–1500 mg/m^2	750–1500 mg/m^2	15–30 mg/kg
Doses/24 h	3 (IV) 5 (oral)	3 (IV) 5 (oral)	3 (IV) 5 (oral)

Am–Bisome Amphotericin B encapsulated in liposome.

	Initial dose	Maximum dose
IV/24 h	1.0 mg/kg	3.0 mg/kg
Doses/24 h	1	1

Note: Initial dose increased daily until maximum tolerated dose reached.

Amikacin Aminoglycoside antibiotic used in serious Gram-negative infections resistant to gentamicin.

	<2 weeks	Child	Adult
IV/24 h	15 mg/kg	15 mg/kg	15 mg/kg
Doses/24 h	2	2	2

Note: The dose of amikacin should be adjusted according to renal function as discussed for gentamicin with appropriate modification. Therapeutic range of amikacin: Trough < 10 mg/l; Peak < 30 mg/l.

Amphotericin B Fungizone antimycotic – dosage for both adults and children.

	Initial dose	Maximum dose
IV/24 h	0.1–0.25 mg/kg	0.6–1.5 mg/kg
Doses/24 h	1	1

Note: Initial dose increased by 0.1–0.25 mg/kg until maximum tolerated dose reached.

Ampicillin Broad-spectrum beta-lactam antibiotic.

	< 1 week	1–4 weeks	Child	Adult
Oral/24 h			40–50 mg/kg	1000–4000 mg
IV/24 h	50–150 mg/kg	75–200 mg/kg	50–300 mg/kg	2000–4000 mg
Doses/24 h	2–3	3–4	4	4

Amoxicillin Broad-spectrum beta-lactam antibiotic.

	Child	Adult
Oral/24 h	25–50 mg/kg	750–3000 mg
Doses/24 h	3	3

Amoxicillin/clavulanate Amoxicillin plus beta-lactamase inhibitor.

	< 3 months	Child	Adult
Oral/24 h		20–40 mg/kg	750–1500 mg
IV/24 h	75 mg/kg	75 mg/kg	3000 mg
Doses/24 h	3	3	3

Note: Dosage expressed as dose of amoxicillin.

Benzylpenicillin Antibiotic of choice for streptococcal infections.

	< 1 week	1–4 weeks	Child	Adult
IV/24 h	50 mg/kg	75 mg/kg	100 mg/kg	1200–2400 mg
Doses/24 h	2	3	4	4

Cefotaxime Third-generation broad-spectrum cephalosporin antibiotic.

	< 2 weeks	Child	Adult
IV/24 h	50–200 mg/kg	100–200 mg/kg	3000–6000 mg
Doses/24 h	2–4	2–4	3

Ceftazidime Third-generation cephalosporin used to treat severe Gram-negative infections.

	< 2 months	Child	Adult
IV/24 h	25–60 mg/kg	30–150 mg/kg	3000–6000 mg
Doses/24 h	2	2–3	2–3

Ceftriaxone Third-generation broad-spectrum cephalosporin antibiotic.

	< 2 weeks	Child	Adult
IV/24 h	50 mg/kg	20–80 mg/kg	1000–4000 mg
Doses/24 h	1	1	1

Cefuroxime Second-generation broad-spectrum cephalosporin antibiotic.

	Child	Adult
IV/24 h	30–100 mg/kg	2250–4500 mg
Doses/24 h	3–4	3

Ciprofloxacin Fluroquinolone antibiotic used for severe infections.

	Child (see note)	Adult
Oral/24 h	7.5–15 mg/kg	500–1500 mg
IV/24 h	5–10 mg/kg	400–800 mg
Doses/24 h	2	2

Notes: (1) Poor cover for Strep. pneumoniae. (2) Not recommended for children (effect on cartilage) unless benefits outweigh risks.

Clarithromycin Macrolide antibiotic.

	Child	Adult
Oral/24 h	15 mg/kg	500–1000 mg
IV/24 h		1000 mg
Doses/24 h	2	2

Clindamycin Lincosamine antibiotic only used for anaerobic infections and staphylococcal abscesses.

	Child	Adult
Oral	12–24 mg/kg	600–1200 mg
IV/24 h	15–40 mg/kg	600–2700 mg
Doses/24 h	4	4

Co-trimoxazole Dosage for general bacterial infections:

	<6 months	Child	Adult
Oral/24 h	24 mg/kg	48 mg/kg	1920 mg
IV/24 h		36 mg/kg	1920 mg
Doses/24 h	2	2	2

Notes: (1) Severe allergy can occur to sulphamethoxazole component. (2) Dosage expressed as co-trimoxazole.

Dosage for pneumocystis infection:

	Adult and child
Oral/24 h	120 mg/kg
IV/24 h	120 mg/kg
Doses/24 h	4

Notes: (1) Severe allergy can occur to sulphamethoxazole component. (2) Dosage expressed as co-trimoxaxole.

Doxycycline Tetracycline antibiotic.

	Adult	
Oral/24 h	100–200 mg	
Doses/24 h	1	

Note: Tetracyclines are not recommended for children because of discoloration of teeth.

Ethambutol Antituberculous antibiotic.

	Adult and child
Oral/24 h	15–25 mg/kg
Doses/24 h	1

Erythromycin Broad-spectrum macrolide antibiotic.

	Infants	**Child**	**Adult**
Oral		20–50 mg/kg	1000–2000 mg
IV/24 h	30–45 mg/kg	50 mg/kg	2000–4000 mg
Doses/24 h	3	4	4

Flucloxacillin Penicillin antibiotic used to treat staphylococcal infections.

	< 2 years	**2–10 years**	**Adult**
Oral/24 h	$\frac{1}{4}$ adult dose	$\frac{1}{2}$ adult dose	1000–2000 mg
IV/24 h	$\frac{1}{4}$ adult dose	$\frac{1}{2}$ adult dose	1000–4000 mg
Doses/24 h	4	4	4

Fluconazole Antifungal agent used to treat systemic candidiasis and cryptococcal infections.

	Child	**Adult**
Oral/24 h	1–6 mg/kg	100–400 mg
IV/24 h	1–6 mg/kg	200–400 mg
Doses/24 h	1	1

Flucytosine Antimycotic.

	Adult and child
Oral/24 h	200 mg/kg
IV/24 h	200 mg/kg
Doses/24 h	4

Foscarnet Antiviral agent used to treat cytomegaloviral infection.

	Adult and child
IV/24 h	21–200 mg/kg
Doses/24 h	2–3

Note: Dosage depends on renal function.

Ganciclovir Antiviral agent used to treat cytomegaloviral infections.

	Adult and child
IV/24 h	10 mg/kg
Doses/24 h	2

Gentamicin Broad-spectrum aminoglycoside antibiotic.

	< 2 weeks	**Child**	**Adult**
IV/24 h	3 mg/kg	6 mg/kg	3–5 mg/kg
Doses/24 h	2	3	3

Note: Dosage of gentamicin is dependent on patient size and renal function:

Creatinine clearance (ml/min)	Maximum adult dose* (mg)	Interval (h)
30–70	80	12
10–30	80	24
5–10	80	48
<5	80	after dialysis

* Reduce 80 mg dose to 60 mg if body weight < 60 kg.

Monitor serum levels of aminoglycosides. In patients with normal renal function the first level should be monitored at the third dose; a trough level should be measured immediately prior to the next dose and a peak level 30 min after IV bolus dose.

Therapeutic range of gentamicin: Trough, < 2 mg/l; Peak, < 10 mg/l.

Samples should be taken twice weekly in patients with normal renal function and daily in those with renal impairment.

Imipenem Broad-spectrum carbapenem antibiotic.

	Child	**Adult**
IV/24 h	60 mg/kg	1500–4000 mg
Doses/24 h	4	3–4

Isoniazid Antituberculous antibiotic.

	Child	**Adult**
Oral/24 h	10 mg/kg	300 mg
Doses/24 h	1	1

Metronidazole Nitromidazole antibiotic used to treat anaerobic infections.

	Child	**Adult**
Oral	22.5 mg/kg	1200 mg
Rectal	22.5 mg/kg	3000 mg
IV/24 h	22.5 mg/kg	1500 mg
Doses/24 h	3	3

Minocycline Tetracycline antibiotic.

	Adult
Oral/24 h	200 mg
Doses/24 h	2

Note: Tetracyclines are not recommended for children because of discoloration of teeth.

Pentamidine Second-line agent to treat pneumocystis infection.

	Adult and child
Nebulization	600 mg
IV/24 h	4 mg/kg
Doses/24 h	1

Piperacillin Beta-lactamase-stable penicillin antibiotic used for severe infections.

	Child	Adult
IV/24 h	50–300 mg/kg	6000–16 000 mg
Doses/24 h	4–6	3–6

Pyrazinamide Antituberculous antibiotic.

	Child	Adult < 50 kg	Adult >50 kg
Oral/24 h	35 mg/kg	1500 mg	2000 mg
Doses/24 h	1	1	1

Rifampicin Antituberculous antibiotic.

	Child	Adult < 50 kg	Adult >50 kg
Oral/24 h	10 mg/kg	450 mg	600 mg
Doses/24 h	1	1	1

Tazocin Piperacillin plus tazobactam – a beta-lactamase inhibitor.

	Adult and child >12 y
IV/24 h	9000–18 000 mg
Doses/24 h	3–4

Ticarcillin Beta-lactamase-stable penicillin.

	Child	Adult
IV/24 h	200–300 mg/kg	15 000–20 000 mg
Doses/24 h	3–4	3–4

Teicoplanin Glycopeptide antibiotic for aerobic and anaerobic Gram-positive bacteria.

	<2 weeks	Child	Adult
IV/24 h	8 mg/kg	6–10 mg/kg	200–400 mg
Doses/24 h	1	1	1

Note: A loading dose may be given as recommended by the company.

Tetracycline Tetracycline antibiotic.

	Adult
Oral/24 h	1000–2000 mg
Doses/24 h	4

Note: Tetracyclines are not recommended for children because of discoloration of teeth.

Tobramycin Broad-spectrum aminoglycoside antibiotic.

	Infant < 1 week	Child	Adult
IV/24 h	4 mg/kg	6–7.5 mg/kg	3–5 mg
Doses/24 h	2	3	3

Note: The dose of tobramycin should be adjusted according to renal function as discussed for gentamicin with appropriate modification.
Therapeutic range of tobramycin: Trough, < 2 mg/l; Peak, < 12 mg/l.

Trimethoprim–Dapsone Combination for treating pneumocystis infection – dosage for adults.

	Dapsone	Trimethoprim
Oral/24 h	100 mg/kg	20 mg/kg
Doses/24 h	1	4

Note: Used to treat patients allergic to sulphamethoxazole.

Vancomycin Glycopeptide antibiotic for aerobic and anaerobic Gram-positive bacteria.

	< 1 week	1–4 weeks	Child	Adult
IV/24 h	20 mg/kg	30 mg/kg	40 mg/kg	2000 mg
Doses/24 h	2	3	4	4

Arguedas AG, Marks MI, Lower respiratory tract infection. In: Engelhard D, Marks MI, Branski D, eds, *Paediatric Infectious Diseases* (Karger: Basel, 1993) 181–98.

Body GP, Milatovic D, Braveny I, *The Antimicrobial Pocket Book* (Freidrich Vieweg: Wiesbaden,1991)

British Thoracic Society and the Public Health Laboratory Service, Community-acquired pneumonia in adults in British Hospitals in 1982–1983: A survey of aetiology, mortality, prognostic features and outcome, *Q J Med* (1987) **239**:195–220.

Douglass JA, Shaw RJ, Respiratory disease associated with HIV infection. In: Brewis RAL, Corrin B, Geddes DM, Gibson GJ, eds, *Respiratory Medicine* 2nd edn (WB Saunders: London,1995) 762–83.

Hopkin JM, Respiratory disease in the immunocompromised host: non-AIDS. In: Brewis RAL, Corrin B, Geddes DM, Gibson GJ, eds, *Respiratory Medicine* 2nd edn (WB Saunders: London, 1995) 784–94.

Macfarlane JT, Acute respiratory infections in adults. In: Brewis RAL, Corrin B, Geddes DM, Gibson GJ, eds, *Respiratory Medicine* 2nd edn (WB Saunders: London, 1995) 705–46.

Woodhead MA, MacFarlane JT, McCracken JS et al, Prospective study of the aetiology and outcome of pneumonia in the community, *Lancet* (1987) **i**: 671–4.

Index

Page numbers in *italic* refer to the illustrations

meconium, 25, 47
prevention, 9
Foscarnet, 63, 72
Fungal pneumonia, 3
  causes, 68
  clinical features,
    19–20
  cysts, 34
  immunocompromised
    host, 11

G

Ganciclovir, 53, 63, 73
Gastro-oesophageal
  reflux, 7, 9, 14, 17
Gentamicin, 45, 60, 61,
  62, 73
Gram-negative bacteria,
  2, 11, 20, 39, 50,
  51, 66, 67
Gram-positive bacteria,
  39, 66, 67

H

Haematology, 30, 41
Haemophilus influenzae,
  2, 48, 66
  antibiotics, 47, 58
  in children, 10, 11,
    45, 46
  in the elderly, 50
  immunization, 8
  nosocomial pneumo-
    nia, 51
  and pleural disease,
    22
  sputum analysis, 40,
    40
Haemorrhage, intraven-
  tricular, 14
Heart disease, 16, 19,
  21, 26, 50
Heart failure, 14, 16, 21,
  27–8, 47, 50
Hernia, congenital
  diaphragmatic, 25
Herpes simplex, 9, 19,
  64
Herpes viruses, 19, 64,
  67
Herpes zoster, 64
Histamine, 29
Histoplasma

capsulatum, 68
Histoplasmosis, 19
Hospital: antibiotics,
  59–65
  hospital-acquired
    pneumonia, 2, 9,
    67
  referral to, 57, 58
Human immunodeficien-
  cy virus (HIV), 1, 5,
  7, 8, 10, 12, 20–1,
  52
Humoral immunodefi-
  ciency, 7
Hyaline membrane
  disease, 25, 47
Hydatid cyst, 26
Hypertension, 50

I

IgA, 7
Imipenem, 61, 62, 73
Immotile cilia, 7
Immunization, 8, 19
Immunocompromised
  host, 2, 9
  antibiotics, 62
  causes of pneumonia,
    11–12
  clinical features, 16
  fungus pneumonia,
    19, 20
  management of pneu-
    monia, 52–3
  Pneumocystis carinii,
    20
  uncommon
    pathogens, 20–1
  virus pneumonia, 19
Immunodeficiency, 7, 8
Immunoglobulins, 7
Immunosuppression, 7
Infants: antibiotics, 60
  causes of pneumonia,
    9–10
  clinical features,
    13–14
  differential diagnosis,
    25
  immunization, 8
  management of pneu-
    monia, 45–7
Influenza, 3, 8, 9, 10–11,
  19, 47–8, 67
Interstitial lung disease,
  26, 50

Interstitial pneumonia, 4,
  5, *6, 37*
Intubation, 7, 9
Invasive procedures,
  41–2
Investigations, 29–42
Ischaemic heart
  disease, 16
Isoniazid, 54, 65, 73

K

Kidney disease, 21
Klebsiella, 3, 10, 20, 67
Klebsiella pneumoniae,
  40, 66

L

Laboratory investiga-
  tions, 36–42
Legionella, 3, 7, 20, 22,
  30, 41, 47, 48, 49,
  52
Legionella pneumophila,
  66
Leukaemia, 53
Leukocytes, 6
Liver disease, 21
Liver function tests, 41
Lobar emphysema, 25
Lobar pneumonia, 3, 4,
  4, 32
Lung abscesses, 17, 34,
  61
Lung function tests, 29,
  31
Lungs, defence mecha-
  nisms, 6–7
Lymphocytic interstitial
  pneumonia, 5, 12
Lymphoma, 26, 34, 53
Lysozyme, 6

M

Macophages, 6
Macrolides, 3, 47
Malignancy, 26, 27, 34,
  50, 53
Management of pneu-
  monia, 43–55,
  56–8
Meconium aspiration,

Coventry University